Intermittent Fasting for Beginners

How to Lose Weight, Boost Energy, and Feel Amazing

Introduction

Intermittent fasting has gained massive popularity over the years and can be deemed a trend in the 21st century. Because intermittent fasting offers the flexibility and freedom to eat what you want, when you want (within your eating window), it has become popular among fitness enthusiasts. The perks of this fasting approach have been recognized over the centuries. Fasting has been a natural and induced method of survival since the existence of hunters and gatherers. During ancient times, it was impossible to find food at times, which is why our ancestors went prolonged periods without eating. This trait has become popular once more and humans have evolved to go for an extended period without eating anything. It is also encouraged due to the numerous health benefits it provides.

Almost every person who aims to lose and maintain weight has tried intermittent fasting at least once in their life. If you want to lose weight and benefit from other health perks with this approach, this book is right up your alley. It will provide information on how intermittent fasting works, why you should do it, who can and shouldn't do it, types of fasting, and how to do it. It has everything you need to know about intermittent fasting as a beginner.

Read on to find out more.

Chapter 1: What is Intermittent Fasting? And Why is it so Popular?

Intermittent fasting is the act of fasting for a specific period, usually between meals. If done correctly, this dieting pattern can provide numerous health benefits and boost weight loss. Even if you are not aiming to lose weight, intermittent fasting assists in maintaining your weight and boosting energy levels. In this type of dieting pattern, an individual goes without eating anything for 12 to 20 hours between meals. Some people even try the 24-hour fast to boost the process. Inexperienced dieters often confuse fasting with starvation. One crucial factor that separates these two – starvation is depriving your body of food for an extended period and is completely involuntary and out of your control. In contrast, fasting is under your control and is conducted only for a specific period.

The phenomenon of intermittent fasting occurs during an absence of food consumption and is carried out over 10 to 12 hours. Some people have this misconception of skipping breakfast and calling it an intermittent fast. If you are one of them, you have got it all wrong. Intermittent fasting includes skipping breakfast, but it needs special consideration about the fasting period, eating right, and breaking the fast without overwhelming the body. If done right, intermittent fasting can offer a myriad of health benefits.

The logic behind intermittent fasting is simple. Your body needs fewer calories to lose weight. By choosing a specific eating window, you are naturally consuming fewer calories because you eat less food. That results in a calorie deficit which, teamed with exercise, can help you to lose weight. Additionally, the changes in hormone levels increase the effect of fat burning. Furthermore, people with busy schedules, which is common nowadays, can easily incorporate intermittent fasting in their regime. They are either too distracted to focus on eating or can easily manage to skip one or two meals. This flexibility is a great factor that inspires and motivates people to follow this fasting approach.

The perks of intermittent fasting are not new to the religious and spiritual world. It is considered common practice to fast for one or more days as a spiritual dedication to God in Islam, Judaism, Hinduism, Christianity, and Buddhism.

One major downside to intermittent fasting is that you are unable to practice and develop mindful eating. Even though it provides a strict window to stick to (which improves self-control), it allows you to eat anything and everything during the window. So, if your eating window falls within the midnight, you will allow yourself to binge on late night snacks and sleep on a heavy stomach. Our body is the least active when we are asleep at night, so by feeding on heavy and greasy food; you are actually increasing the chances of gaining weight. Also, since you are eating by the clock, you have to eat, even if you are not hungry.

Even though your appetite follows a pattern and tells you when you are hungry, you can still experience some daily changes due to the changes in hormones, exercise routine, stress levels, and environmental factors. However, you can note your hunger pattern every day and try to prepare a schedule accordingly. All in all, intermittent fasting does provide numerous health benefits but also results in an inappropriate eating habit.

The Popularity of Intermittent Fasting

Intermittent fasting has been approached as a practice for centuries. However, it was never structured as a dieting pattern before. With time, experts realized the health benefits of this diet and decided to experiment with it. The dieting approach became more popular in the 21st century, particularly in the last decade, when the TV documentary 'Eat Fast, Live Longer' was released by BBC journalist Michael Mosley in 2012. The next release, which was a book called 'The Fast Diet,' enhanced the concept of intermittent fasting and brought it to the limelight. Several other releases on the same topic pushed intermittent fasting as one of the top dieting approaches of the decade. Some of these notable releases include 'The 5:2 Diet' by journalist Kate Harrison, in 2013, and 'The Obesity Code' by Jason Fung, MD, in 2016.

Many celebrities and prominent figures tried this dieting approach and found it to be successful, which furthered its popularity. Slowly and steadily, intermittent fasting became a household name due to its flexibility of fasting, freedom of eating whatever you want, not counting or tracking macros and calories, and still losing weight. Many people now consider this approach as their 'savior' and follow it religiously. There are many online and offline communities of 'fasters' who share their experience and give tips to beginners.

Chapter 2: How Does it Affect Your Body?

There have been several debates related to the health risks of intermittent fasting. Irrespective of the numerous health benefits, intermittent fasting is still considered to be a fad at times and is always at the peak of controversy in the dieting world. In this chapter, we will take a look at how intermittent fasting affects your body based on facts.

Ideally, intermittent fasting is successful when your body starts burning its fat reserves in the absence of food and energy. The effects of intermittent fasting are so prolific that it has been around for centuries. In fact, this ancient practice enabled humans to fast for hours and days at a stretch without facing detrimental health issues.

Here is how intermittent fasting works – When you eat food, your body stores the extra energy as reserves that can be used in the absence of calories and food; this phenomenon of energy storage is carried out by the hormone called insulin. As soon as you eat, insulin levels in your body spike, which then acts to store energy in two different ways - the production of glucose from consumed carbs and the other is the storage of fat in the liver and other parts of the body. In the first process, the extra glycogen that is converted from carbs is stored in the liver and muscles to be used as energy. The second process is known as de-novo lipogenesis when the liver converts excess glucose into fat, which is then stored in the liver and other fat deposits around the body. Since there is no limit to the creation and storage of fat, the process keeps on converting glycogen into fat whenever we overeat or feed more calories to the body.

When we do not eat food or fail to provide sufficient calories to our body, the insulin levels drop. It instructs our body to use the stored glycogen and fat as energy. At the same time, our blood glucose levels also drop, which is when the reserve energy helps. After all the glucose is used up as energy, the body begins using the fat deposits to produce energy. The more fat it burns, the more weight we lose. If you increase your fasting period, your body will use up more energy, which will ultimately burn more fat.

How it Affects Cells and Hormones

Fasting also affects your body at a hormonal and cellular level. Your body releases certain hormones to enable your body to use stored fat as energy. It is also known that your cells undergo an expression in their genes and start to repair the damaged parts.

These are the hormonal and cellular changes that take place in one's body during intermittent fasting including:

• **Insulin:** In the absence of food, insulin levels drop, and the sensitivity to insulin improves. This is beneficial as your body is then able to access stored body fat more easily.

• **Human Growth Hormone (HGH):** HGH levels increase exponentially, almost by 5 times. With increased HGH levels, you benefit from faster fat loss, and you gain more muscle.

• **Changes in Gene Expression:** With these changes, your cells improve their power to fight against diseases and provide longevity.

• **Cellular Repair:** Your cells improve activity during the fasting stage to repair or remove old protein blocks from the cells, which is also known as autophagy.

How it Affects Women

The topic of intermittent fasting for women has witnessed numerous debates to date. While some experts claim that women shouldn't follow intermittent fasting to lose weight, others say that it is absolutely safe. During intermittent fasting, your body undergoes a significant change in hormonal and cellular levels. When faced with hormonal changes in their bodies women can face several issues, such as irregular menstrual cycles, acne, weight loss or gain, hair loss, etc.

Let's take a look at three studies conducted on men and women to compare the effects of intermittent fasting on both genders –

1. A study was conducted on 8 men and 8 women (non-obese), where these candidates went through three weeks of intermittent fasting. It was found that the insulin levels were untethered in women, whereas the glucose levels changed with every meal. On the other hand, all men showed slight changes (reduction) in insulin levels and no change in glucose levels.

2. Another study conducted on 11 women who underwent a 72-hour fast concluded a major change in their metabolic responses. There was an increase in the cortisol level, which is the stress hormone, and advanced the central circadian clock, which is responsible for operating and designing our sleeping pattern.

3. A third study conducted on 8 women with a 72-hour fast concluded that there was no significant change in their menstrual cycles despite facing changes in the metabolic responses in the follicular phase.

Source: https://www.nerdfitness.com/blog/a-beginners-guide-to-intermittent-fasting/ (PubMed Archives)

These studies show that glucose and insulin responses were more positive in men than in women, which says that intermittent fasting is more effective for weight loss in men. Other sources say that intermittent fasting and its caloric restriction can cause reproductive issues, irregular menstrual cycles, increased stress levels, plausible early menopause, etc. However, there is no substantial research regarding this, and we need more data to back it up.

There appears to be a significant difference in the response to intermittent fasting in men and women, at least for some people. Also, it seems a bit risky for women to follow intermittent fasting as a part of their overall lifestyle. However, every person is different and shows varied effects from intermittent fasting. Hence, it all boils down to the individual's response to this fasting approach.

Lastly, if you are a woman who is planning on taking this fasting route, stay away from this option if you are experiencing one of these issues or conditions –

- When you are pregnant

- If you have a history of any eating disorder

- If you suffer from chronic stress

- If you have never exercised or followed a diet before

- If you have trouble sleeping

- If you are suffering from irregular menstrual cycles

If you still want to lose weight and burn fat, eat right, and exercise regularly to lose extra pounds the regular way.

Can you Pair Intermittent Fasting with Keto Diet?

Individuals who are keen on losing weight at a faster pace often combine intermittent fasting with keto. The keto diet is a low-carb, high-fat diet that produces ketones from fat to use as energy, eventually boosting weight loss. When your body is deprived of carbs, it fails to produce glucose and glycogen, which is used as energy to carry out functions in your body. When you deprive your body of food during intermittent fasting, it enters into mild ketosis, which is an effective way to kick-start your weight loss journey.

Intermittent fasting, in a way, also takes a similar approach, which is why it is often paired with keto. How exactly? When you are allowed to eat in your eating window during intermittent fasting, you should replace your regular meals with high-fat and low-carb meals. The carb content is usually limited to around 20 to 50 grams per day. When you eat a keto meal, you are putting your body into ketosis, and when you are fasting, you are sustaining the ketosis for a prolonged period, hence enhancing the fat burning process.

However, the keto diet in itself is a challenging approach to lose weight. When paired with intermittent fasting, it can be extremely difficult. So, before you decide to combine these two, make sure that you are already acquainted with and are used to intermittent fasting. One important consideration in this combination is the macronutrients. While you don't have to count macronutrients on intermittent fasting, you should pay attention to the number of carbs and fat content in keto. It is essential to trigger ketosis, which will burn more fat.

Chapter 3: Pros and Cons of Intermittent Fasting

This type of fasting comes with several pros and cons.

Pros

1. Weight Loss

As we know, our body uses up fat deposits as energy when it is deprived of food. The longer you fast, the more fat you burn, which will eventually cut pounds from your body mass. Intermittent fasting is one of the easiest ways to lose weight; it allows you to eat whatever you like and still boosts weight loss. Most people approach this method of intermittent fasting as it is a powerful tool to lose weight and burn fat. It also considers your routine and provides flexibility. With reduced meals, you are already cutting back on calories, which is another reason why intermittent fasting is effective in losing weight. Additionally, your hormone levels fluctuate, which assists in weight loss. Norepinephrine or noradrenaline is a fat-burning hormone that increases in functionality during intermittent fasting. As such, more fat is burned and more weight is lost.

2. Prolongs Life

Intermittent fasting is known to prolong one's life and enhances the longevity of cells. The cells in our body are triggered during intermittent fasting and function to repair and remove damaged protein; this activity revives the cells and improves your health. It is also known that when people face prolonged calorie restrictions, they undergo a boost in their lifespan and lower the risk of certain diseases, the most common being cancer.

3. No Need to Count Calories

When losing weight on a diet, people need to count calories regularly, which can be quite frustrating at times. You have to use a tracking app and note every meal in it or maintain a fitness journal to track your calories. It is highly likely that you will forget or be too busy to track a meal. With intermittent fasting, you merely have to track the fasting period and pay attention to the eating window, which is much easier than counting calories. To make it even easier, you can plan your meals ahead and count the calories beforehand. Since intermittent fasting doesn't require accurate counting or little counting of calories, you can just note the calories mentioned on the packet of food or use a smartphone. Even if you can't do it, don't fret. Intermittent fasting automatically offers calorie restriction as it allows just 1 or 2 meals in a day, hence keeping the count low.

4. No Need to Count Macronutrients

Just like calories, counting macronutrients is not required during intermittent fasting. Also, like some nutrition plans, you don't have to limit certain macronutrients. For instance, keto diets impose a restriction on carb intake, where you should consume only 20 to 50 grams of carbs in a day to lose weight. Similarly, some diets ask you to lower your fat intake to improve health and lose weight. All these diets suggest that you adopt a new way of eating and cooking. You might have to find and include some new recipes or ingredients to accommodate the needs of these diets.

However, with intermittent fasting, there is no need to restrict macronutrients. You can eat whatever you like and prefer to cook. You can follow intermittent fasting while traveling or going to new restaurants, given that you are following the fasting and eating window. Since you are allowed to eat anything you like, you will also have no cravings.

5. Reduces Cholesterol and Combats other Health Issues

Intermittent fasting is known to promote other health benefits, too, with lowered cholesterol being one of the main advantages. Apart from cholesterol, the levels of triglycerides and LDL are reduced, too. Along with this, intermittent fasting also reduces inflammation and prevents certain chronic issues related to age. All this without affecting the person's physical activity levels.

Cons

1. Constipation

This is one of the most common side effects of intermittent fasting, especially if followed at a widened window. Naturally, less eating means less excretion. Even though it isn't a big concern, you should consult a general practitioner when you suffer from abdominal discomfort, bloating, or pain. To ease the negative effect, you can add magnesium supplements in your diet or use standard laxatives. Another way to cure constipation is by adding more fibrous food in your diets such as lentils, beans, bananas, and dark vegetables. Keep drinking water to cure constipation further. It is a common side effect in the initial stages of fasting, but once your body gets used to the new way of eating, you will no longer suffer from this issue.

2. Hunger Pangs

It is safe to assume that when your body is deprived of food for a longer window, it will make gurgling sounds, and you might also suffer from painful hunger pangs. However, this is only a temporary wave and will pass within an hour or two. All you have to do is learn to control your temptations during this phase. You don't have to worry about hunger pangs being a permanent issue during fasting as it usually passes within no time. As your body adapts to the new way of eating, it will also tolerate hunger in the absence of food; you just need to give yourself some time to adapt to the sudden change. Many intermittent fasting beginners have reported that hunger increases by day 2 and becomes almost intolerable. However, it gradually recedes by day 3 or 4 and eventually vanishes. By now, your body knows that it needs to feed on the extra fat deposits in your body due to the absence of food, which will control your hunger pangs and let you get through the day.

Furthermore, to keep hunger pangs away, add a lot of protein in your diet. At the same time, keep drinking water to avoid kidney issues due to increased protein intake. Fiber is important, too, so eat more fiber to keep your stomach full for a longer period. It will also increase bowel movement and avoid constipation. By filling up on protein and fiber, you can avoid hunger pangs in the morning, and it will assist you in getting to lunch.

3. Possible Lean Body Mass Loss

Several debates about the loss of muscle along with fat due to intermittent fasting are resurfacing. Most overweight dieters will burn fat during the fasting phase. However, leaner individuals might face a reduced metabolic rate along with loss of lean mass. They don't have many fat deposits in their body to burn, which is why the body will directly target the muscle mass because the building blocks of proteins, which are the excess amino acids are broken down to be used as energy. However, if there is some fat in your body to be used up, your muscles wouldn't be targeted unless it's an emergency. Hence, this is not a major concern.

4. Might be Stressful

Even though this fasting approach is flexible and suited to most schedules, it can, at times, be very stressful for some people. For most people, it is a blessing, whereas, for some, it is a huge bane. The restrictive calorie window is difficult for some people to abide by, especially for those who are unable to follow the rules. Also, people who frequently travel to different places and in various time zones can simply not follow this approach. It is too difficult and stressful to keep track of the time zones and track your meals. This additional stress can result in additional weight gain, which is the opposite of our main goal if you don't like the thought of waiting for the clock to strike to have your meal or that 'permission grant' to eat eventually, think twice before taking up intermittent fasting.

5. Chances of Hypoglycemia

One of the common downsides of intermittent fasting is low blood sugar levels, which is also known as hypoglycemia. This health issue occurs due to skipping meals or eating less food. Individuals who have diabetes and are on insulin medication often suffer from hypoglycemia, but it can also happen to people without diabetes in some cases. Intermittent fasting should be avoided if suffering from this condition as it can cause dizziness, nausea, paleness, sweating, blurred vision, and uneasiness. Individuals with thyroid issues should also avoid intermittent fasting, as they are more prone to hypoglycemia.

Chapter 4: Different Clocks of Intermittent Fasting

As you know, the effects of intermittent fasting only work when you provide a gap of at least 12 or more hours.

The choice of period gaps depends on the individual and varies from person to person. Different people use different clocks depending on their schedule, self-control, and health.

There are two main types of intermittent fasting – shorter fasts (with a window of fewer than 24 hours) and longer fasts (with a window of more than 24 hours). Both of these fasting types further possess varied fasting windows, which provide similar health benefits but different schedules.

Shorter Fasts – Less than 24 hours

As the name suggests, this type of fast is carried out in shorter intervals and provides a person with full flexibility and the ability to adjust the plan according to their schedule. These can be conducted more frequently but should be done only for a few days with regular intervals. If you want to continue pursuing a short intermittent fast, you should do it under medical supervision.

These fasting windows are the most popular in shorter fasts –

1. 12:12

This type of fast gives you a 12-hour eating bracket and a 12-hour fasting window in a day. You need to eat all meals within this 12-hour window and go without eating in the next 12 hours. It is the safest and offers a great start to your intermittent fasting practice. Once you get used to it, you can then switch to a longer fasting window. However, this is the least effective of all fasting types as it provides lesser time for your body to burn fat. Since it is easy to follow, you can follow it every day without much trouble. A typical eating schedule would be eating from 9 am to 9 pm, which will consist of three meals in a day, with or without snacks.

Why is this the least effective clock of all? When you eat dinner and wake up the next morning, your body still has carbs and glucose stored from the previous meal. Your body will burn these remaining deposits to gain energy for a few more hours after you wake up. The gap between consuming an average-sized meal and using up the last deposits of carbs as energy is approximately 10 to 12 hours. So, as soon as your body uses up the last deposits of glucose and switches to fat burning for energy, you are consuming another meal in the morning. By doing so, your body is regaining more carbs and glucose, which is primarily burned as energy. So, even before you give your body a decent chance to burn fat and use it up, you are feeding it more food. Hence, this approach is best to begin practicing intermittent fasting and to maintain weight.

2. 14:10

This type of fast gives you a 10-hour eating bracket and a 14-hour fasting window in a day. You need to eat all meals within this 10-hour window and go without eating for the next 14 hours. Once you are acquainted with the 12:12 fasting bracket, you can then increase the fasting bracket to 2 more hours. This bracket is also easy to follow and offers similar health benefits, and you can follow it every day with ease. A typical eating schedule would be eating from 9 am to 7 pm, which will consist of three meals a day. With a 14-hour window, your body will get a few more hours to burn fat compared to the 12:12 fasting approach, making it an effective option.

3. 16:8

This type of fast gives you an 8-hour eating bracket and a 16-hour fasting window in a day. You need to eat all meals within this 8-hour window and go without eating for the next 16 hours of your day. By this stage, it will get a bit difficult. However, it is recommended to practice with the 12:12 and 14:10 fasting periods before jumping onto this fasting period. A typical eating schedule would be eating from 11 am to 7 pm, which will consist of two to three meals a day. You can either skip breakfast or squeeze it in this period. This type of fast needs to be followed for a few days with a break. In the 16:8 fasting approach, your body gets 16 hours to use up all carbs and glucose deposits and also burn fat to use up as energy, which accelerates the weight loss process while not letting you starve.

4. 18:6

This type of fast gives you a 6-hour eating bracket and an 18-hour fasting window a day. You need to eat all meals within this 6-hour window and go without eating for the next 18 hours of your day. It is also a super effective and a safer option to reap almost similar health benefits like you would from the 20:4 fasting window. A typical eating schedule would be eating from 1 pm to 7 pm, which will consist of two to three meals a day. You need to skip breakfast and stick to two heavy meals and a small snack in this period. This fasting window cannot be followed regularly over a prolonged period and needs a break of a few days before you begin the next cycle. In the 18:6 fasting approach, your body gets 18 hours to use up all carbs and glucose deposits and also burns fat to use up as energy, which makes it a better option than the 16:8 approach. However, it is more difficult than the ones mentioned above.

5. 20:4

This type of fast gives you a 4-hour eating bracket and a 20-hour fasting window a day. You need to eat all meals within this 4-hour window and go without eating for the next 20 hours. It is the most difficult short fast that one can follow for a few days. You need a lot of determination and practice from the previous fasting windows to follow this type of fast. It is the most effective fasting type and provides maximum fat burning compared to its counterparts. In this fasting approach, your body gets 20 hours to use up all carbs and glucose deposits and also burns fat to use up as energy, which is an extremely prolonged period. This approach is the fastest way to lose weight through intermittent fasting daily.

Even though it requires a lot of self-control and determination to follow this type of fast, it is easier to continue once your body gets acquainted with it. A typical eating schedule would be eating from 3 pm to 7 pm or 1 pm to 5 pm, which will consist of two heavy meals in a day. If you want, you can stick to just one heavy meal and a light snack as it is unlikely to get hungry within 2 hours. This fasting window cannot be followed regularly over a prolonged period and needs a break of a few days before you begin the next cycle as it reduces nutritional content in your body. If you want to continue it for a prolonged period, you should seek medical supervision.

To make it easier, begin with the 12:12 fast. Take a break of one week and extend the fasting period by 2 hours to switch to the 14:10 fasting window. Take a break again in the next week and extend it again by 2 hours. Repeat this process until you successfully reach the 20:4 fasting window. Most people think that it is impossible to achieve such a feat. However, according to several experienced dieters, they began with no hope but are successfully following the 20:4 fasting window regularly. They have also noted the health effects and positive changes through this extended gap.

Longer Fasts – More than 24 Hours

In this category, the fasts are prolonged and conducted over 24 hours or more on an extended and continuous basis. These are a bit more difficult than shorter fasts but provide better results.

These fasting windows are the most popular in longer fasts –

1. 24 Hours

As the name suggests, this fast is where you go without eating for 24 hours at a stretch. This approach is also called the 'Eat Stop Eat' method of fasting. You break the fast by eating during dinner time and fast again until the next dinner. Some people plan and adjust their meals according to their schedules and preferences. For instance, you can keep the fasting window from breakfast to breakfast or from lunch to lunch. Whatever it is you choose, make sure that there is a 24-hour window between your meals; this approach of fasting is also known as one meal a day or OMAD fasting. You need a gap of two to three days between each fast. Take a break of a few weeks before you begin another cycle. Stick to low-carb and healthy meals during the break to avoid regaining body weight.

2. 36 Hours

This is a wilder approach to fasting and is more difficult than fasting for 24 hours. In a 36-hour fast, you fast for the whole day and do not eat until the next main meal. For instance, if you eat dinner on day 1, you skip the entire day 2 and only eat again at breakfast on day 3. You can choose the meals and schedule this plan according to your preference. Just make sure that there is a 36-hour fasting window between the meals. Since this kind of fasting, the approach isn't really suited to most people, consult your general practitioner before you begin fasting.

3. 5:2

This is a rather popular fasting approach due to the immense scientific support it has garnered over the years. In this type of fasting, you eat regularly for five days and fast for 2 days. However, you are allowed to eat up to 500 calories during these two fasting days. You can either spread the calories throughout the day or consume them all in one meal; this approach is easier to follow and has a lot of health benefits too. The best part is, you can do this every week and make it a part of your lifestyle.

4. Alternate Days

This is a similar approach to the 5:2 fasting style, but the only difference is that you need to eat 500 calories every alternate day in a week. So, your day 1 will be normal eating, day 2 will be eating 500 calories spread throughout the day or in a single meal, day 3 will, again, be normal eating, day 4 will be consuming 500 calories, and so on. This alternate day fasting method provides health benefits, boosts weight loss, and does not overwhelm your body with the new changes.

5. Extended Fasts

This approach of fasting wants you to fast at an extended period, usually around or more than 48 hours. It is the most challenging fasting style of them all and thus requires you to check with your general practitioner first. This fast is not recommended for individuals with existing health conditions. Since you are not consuming any food for 2 days, your body will be devoid of nutrients. Hence, it is advised to take a multivitamin every day to fulfill nutrition requirements. Although the recommended period of an extended fast is 48 hours, some people have tried fasting for over 7 to 14 days - the highest record is 382 days. Fasting for more than 14 days is not advised as it could lead to the re-feeding syndrome, which is the condition of your body during the re-shifting of electrolytes and fluids when food is consumed after a long time.

Chapter 5: Create a Plan

Before we learn how to create an intermittent fasting plan, let's talk about the meals. Some experts emphasize the importance of skipping breakfast for intermittent fasting and to achieve the fasting window, whereas others suggest skipping dinner. So, what's the real deal?

For the sole purpose of achieving a larger fasting window, you can skip any of these meals for your body to use up fat as energy. However, it is known that skipping breakfast provides a longer bracket to sustain the fast and allows your body to burn more fat because your hunger level is at the lowest in the morning and will make it easier for you to skip breakfast. Most of us get hungry at midnight, despite having a large meal for dinner. For this reason, it is safer to eat dinner and skip breakfast.

However, if you prefer eating breakfast over dinner, you can take this approach, too.

Once you have sorted out your meals and learned about the foods you can eat, you should know when and how you can break your fast. As the clock strikes, the fasting window closes, and the time to eat finally arrives. Some people go all in and indulge in greasy, unhealthy food, and overeat. This approach is unhealthy and should preferably be dealt with gently. Eating too much, all at once, is harmful to your body. You can suffer from bloating, gas, and stomach ache.

Breaking Your Fast

To break your fast, begin gently; start with a small snack and wait for at least an hour to eat your bigger meal. In fact, the bigger your fasting window is, the longer you should wait to switch to the bigger meal. Occasional indulgences are welcomed but do not overfeed your body with heavy meals; this will delay your weight loss results, and all your efforts will be in vain. Once you get into the fasting routine, your body will adapt to the new style of eating, without feeling overwhelmed.

Most importantly, avoid binge eating. As we've been emphasizing the importance of calorie count, binge eating can ruin the health effects of intermittent fasting. Do your best to ward off binge eating behavior. There is no point in fasting for 16 hours and then binging on 5,000 calories in the remaining 8 hours of your day. It will have an opposite effect on your body, and you might end up gaining more weight. This is particularly challenging for people who eat at regular intervals without understanding their bodies during hunger.

How to Get Started

Now, it is time to design an approach that suits your needs. Follow these steps to design a plan that sticks with you for longer.

1. Choose a type of fast that is preferable for you.

2. Choose the length of the fasting window (you can begin with a smaller window initially and increase it gradually).

3. Begin your fast. If you are unable to sustain it on day 1, go back to your normal routine and try it again. Put in your maximum effort before you decide to quit. By sustaining it for 1 or 2 days, you can successfully incorporate it into your regime. However, if you do not feel well, then go back to normal eating.

4. Keep yourself busy to stay distracted and keep cravings away. Keep drinking water before, during, and after your fasting window.

5. Break your fast with a fruit or a light snack and wait for some time before you eat a heavy meal.

6. Repeat this process every day.

Typical Week Plan

After looking at what a typical day will look like on intermittent fasting, let's take a look at what a typical week will look like. We begin with the 12:12 hour on day 1 and gradually increase our fasting window by the end of the week.

Day 1 – 12:12 Approach

This is the first day of your intermittent fasting and the most important. It is crucial to stay committed and motivated on day 1 as it will unravel your determination to continue following this fast for the rest of the week. On day 1, we will skip dinner and have other meals as usual.

Here is a typical healthy meal plan to get you started.

7:00 am – Oatmeal with cinnamon and banana slices or scrambled eggs

10:00 am – Handful of nuts and seeds

1:00 to 2:00 pm – Grilled or sautéed veggies with quinoa or rice and a portion of meat

4:00 pm – An apple or any other fruit

7:00 pm – A large meat or fish portion with more veggies and a side dish

Essentially, sticking to healthy meals and ingredients can increase the pace of weight loss and help you get to your main goal faster. You should have a heavy dinner to get you through the night without trouble and sustain hunger until breakfast. If you get hungry at night, do not give up. Try to calm your hunger and cravings with lukewarm water or green tea. A cup of calming herbal tea works wonders. Another tip to get you through this temptation battle is brushing your teeth. The minty taste in your mouth will satiate your cravings, and you won't feel like eating anything once you have brushed your teeth. It's a great way of saying that you are done eating for the day. Lastly, if nothing works, go to sleep. It will be a bit difficult to sleep it off, but you need to train your mind and body to it. You have eaten enough all day; it is time to stop and sleep.

Congratulations, you have successfully experienced intermittent fasting on your first day and fulfilled the 12:12 approach.

Day 2- Delaying Breakfast

After having achieved the 12:12 ratio of fasting, it is time to take it up a notch. We will try to fast for a longer period on day 2. It's 7:00 am again, which means that your 12-hour fasting window is finished. To continue the 12:12 fasting approach, you can eat breakfast at 7:00 am on day 2. However, since we are trying to extend our fasting window, you should delay eating breakfast for a longer period. Instead of waking up and grabbing something to eat before rushing to your workplace, aim at eating breakfast only when it is convenient. Just sip on some water, coffee, or tea instead of eating right away.

Reach your workplace, mark your presence, and settle in first. Plan your day, and organize your tasks. Basically, follow your morning routine as usual and get things in order first. If you are at home, follow your morning routine, do some necessary cleaning, and plan your day before you eat breakfast as you'd normally do. The point is, don't try to sneak breakfast in; instead, enjoy it without any distractions and by taking your time.

Here is how your day 2 would look like –

10:00 am – By 10:00 am, you will have time to eat your breakfast. It is a 3-hour delay compared to day 1, which increases your fasting period. If possible, you can also try to increase the window by having breakfast an hour later. If not, you can also eat it at 9:00 am. The bottom line is, try to delay your breakfast on day 2 as long as you can. A 2-hour delay is also appreciated.

2:00 pm – Grilled or sautéed veggies with quinoa or rice and a portion of meat (you can add other healthy recipes too)

4:00 pm – An apple or any other fruit

7:00 pm – A large meat or fish portion with more

veggies and a side dish

The timings for lunch and snacks are just as tentative; you can eat according to your schedule and appetite. Just make sure that you finish your dinner by 7:00 pm again, and as day 1. If you feel hungry around 10:00 to 11:00 pm, try to curb your appetite with some curbing tea or sleep it off. We have to get through the night without eating.

Day 3 – No Snacking

By the morning of day 3, you will have achieved a 15-hour fast (given you stick to the 10:00 am breakfast time). On day 3, we will follow the same routine as day 2. The only difference is that we will avoid snacks.

Here are some tips for sustaining hunger during the snacking time, which will get you to dinner without much hassle:

• Tweak your eating time. Since you won't get any snacks at the usual 4:00 pm snacking time, you can delay lunchtime by an hour or two. So, instead of eating lunch at 2:00 pm, which is your usual time, you should move it to 3:00 or 3:30 pm. You will then get hungry directly at 7 pm, which is your dinner time.

• Drink water. At times, our body misinterprets thirst for food cravings. Whenever you feel hungry, drink some water. If the craving goes away, it merely means that you were thirsty. Water curbs appetite, so keep a water bottle handy and drink as much water as you can. We are aiming for at least 3 to 4 liters in a day. It will also calm you down when you are stressed, worried, bored, or anxious.

• Keep yourself distracted. If you are at your workplace, you can easily distract yourself by taking on more tasks or immersing yourself in your work. If you are at home, play with your dog or read a book. Do something productive to feel good about yourself. By distracting yourself, you won't pay much attention to hunger and food, hence keeping yourself from feeding on snacks.

Once you can get past snacking time, it is now time to eat dinner when the clock strikes 7:00 pm. On day 3, you are following the same 15-hour fasting window as day 2; the only difference is the elimination of snacks; this creates a calorie-deficit and burns more fat.

Day 4 – No Breakfast

Day 4 is a real challenge. On this day, you will skip breakfast. It sounds difficult, but all you have to do is wait one more hour to have your morning meal. For instance, if you are eating breakfast at 10:00 am, you just have to wait one more hour to eat your first meal at 11:00 am. In reality, this will be your lunch. It will feel a bit weird to adapt to this new system of eating lunch earlier than usual, but you will swear by this routine in the long run.

Your day 4 meal plan will look like this –

11:00 am – Grilled or sautéed veggies with quinoa or rice and a portion of meat (you can add other healthy recipes too)

4:00 pm – An apple or any other fruit

7:00 pm – A large meat or fish portion with more veggies and a side dish

To continue waiving off your hunger pangs –

- Distract yourself by accomplishing more tasks.

- Drink water when you feel hungry.

- Practice mindful eating, i.e., only eating when you are truly hungry and not while doing something else.

- Constantly motivating yourself to achieve the goal.

These tips and tricks should get you through the day. On day 4, you will have managed eating lunch as your first meal. Eat your snack in the middle of the day so that it sustains you until dinner. Eat dinner at 7 pm. By this time, your body will train itself to sustain hunger past 7:00 pm, and it will be easier for you to control your hunger until bedtime. By the end of day 4, you will successfully achieve a 16-hour fasting window.

Day 5 – 16-Hour Fast with no Snack

Your day 5 will look similar to day 4; the only difference is that you will skip the snack. By this time, you will successfully endure the 16:8 fasting approach, which is the most popular intermittent fasting method. It is easy to follow and offers numerous health benefits. This approach was popularized by the belief that most people tend to skip breakfast or do not prefer eating in the morning; it is also easier for most people to skip breakfast. You only have 8 hours to eat and just two meals to feed on.

Your day 5 meal plan will look like this –

11:00 am – A portion of meat or fish with salad and heavy salad dressing. You can also switch it to whole wheat pasta or healthy turkey meat burgers. Make sure that your meal is heavy to sustain you until dinner.

7:00 pm – A large meat or fish portion with more veggies and a side dish

Make sure that you keep your nutrient intake in check. Since you are reducing your food intake to only 2 meals, your body might lack some essential nutrients. Hence, it is necessary to keep track of nutrients. To do this, note the quantity and nutritional quality of every ingredient you are using. You can use a tracking app to measure it for accuracy. If you feel that your meals are lacking certain essential nutrients (which you should not), take multivitamins that cover the deficiency. However, it is advised to consult your doctor before taking this step.

Day 6

If you are working on day 6 as well, it would be easier to sustain the fast. Repeat the same cycle as day 5 to achieve a 16-hour fast and 8-hour eating window; this will boost weight loss and burn more fat. If you are not working, it is wiser to stick to a normal routine unless you can fast the entire day.

Day 7

On day 7, you can relax and enjoy the day off. It is time to give your body some rest. You can eat whatever you like on this day.

Repeat the entire weekly cycle once again. If you want, you can take some time off between fasting cycles. If these timings don't suit you, you can create a window between 8:00 am to 4:00 pm or 1:00 pm to 9:00 pm. Irrespective of the timings, you have to make sure that you are eating within 8 hours and fasting for the rest of 16 hours a day. Take a look at your schedule and set the timings accordingly. At the same time, make sure that you are following the same timings throughout the week to keep things inflow. For this, you will have to consider your weekly schedule instead of your daily routine. Stick to what works best for you.

It is essential to keep practicing this fasting routine and incorporate it into your regime as a part of your lifestyle. Since it is an easy way to lose weight and sustain health, intermittent fasting can be followed as a regular part of your routine. It will seem a bit difficult initially, but with practice and consistency, you can seamlessly incorporate it as a part of your lifestyle.

Once you can follow the 16:8 method with ease, all your cycles should consist of the same hours and fasting windows.

To make it even easier, stick this schedule on your bedside table or work desk to keep track of your 16:8 fasting approach daily.

Leangains Method for Daily Intermittent Fasting

Sunday

Midnight to 4 am: Sleeping and fasting

4 am to 8 am: Sleeping and fasting

8 am to Noon: Fasting

Noon to 4 pm: Eating

4 pm to 8 pm: Eating

8 pm to Midnight: Fasting

Monday

Midnight to 4 am: Sleeping and fasting

4 am to 8 am: Sleeping and fasting

8 am to Noon: Fasting

Noon to 4 pm: Eating

4 pm to 8 pm: Eating

8 pm to Midnight: Fasting

Tuesday

Midnight to 4 am: Sleeping and fasting

4 am to 8 am: Sleeping and fasting

8 am to Noon: Fasting

Noon to 4 pm: Eating

4 pm to 8 pm: Eating

8 pm to Midnight: Fasting

Wednesday

Midnight to 4 am: Sleeping and fasting

4 am to 8 am: Sleeping and fasting

8 am to Noon: Fasting

Noon to 4 pm: Eating

4 pm to 8 pm: Eating

8 pm to Midnight: Fasting

Thursday

Midnight to 4 am: Sleeping and fasting

4 am to 8 am: Sleeping and fasting

8 am to Noon: Fasting

Noon to 4 pm: Eating

4 pm to 8 pm: Eating

8 pm to Midnight: Fasting

Friday

Midnight to 4 am: Sleeping and fasting

4 am to 8 am: Sleeping and fasting

8 am to Noon: Fasting

Noon to 4 pm: Eating

4 pm to 8 pm: Eating

8 pm to Midnight: Fasting

Saturday

Midnight to 4 am: Sleeping and fasting

4 am to 8 am: Sleeping and fasting

8 am to Noon: Fasting

Noon to 4 pm: Eating

4 pm to 8 pm: Eating

8 pm to Midnight: Fasting

By looking at this schedule, you can easily keep track of your daily eating habits and achieve the best possible results. As suggested, it is wiser to get started with intermittent fasting by following it once a week or once a month. Once you get the hang of it, you can follow weekly schedules and take breaks in between. For example, week 1 of a month will be fasting, and you can take a break in week 2. Continue the cycle by following it in week 3 and taking a break in week 4. It will give your body some time to adapt and boost health benefits at the same time. This approach of occasional fasting is known to provide more health benefits compared to regular fasting. However, you might want to take a look at the calorie count as it will increase during your breaks. Apart from weight loss, you can still gain other health benefits.

To follow a monthly plan more effectively, stick this

schedule on your bedside table or work desk to keep track of your 16:8 fasting approach for the entire week.

Weekly Intermittent Fasting Schedule

Sunday

Midnight to 4 am: Sleeping and fasting

4 am to 8 am: Sleeping and fasting

8 am to Noon: Eating

Noon to 4 pm: Eating

4 pm to 8 pm: Eating

8 pm to Midnight: Eating

Monday

Midnight to 4 am: Sleeping and fasting

4 am to 8 am: Sleeping and fasting

8 am to Noon: Eating

Noon to 4 pm: Fasting

4 pm to 8 pm: Fasting

8 pm to Midnight: Fasting

Tuesday

Midnight to 4 am: Sleeping and fasting

4 am to 8 am: Sleeping and fasting

8 am to Noon: Fasting

Noon to 4 pm: Eating

4 pm to 8 pm: Eating

8 pm to Midnight: Eating

Wednesday

Midnight to 4 am: Sleeping and fasting

4 am to 8 am: Sleeping and fasting

8 am to Noon: Eating

Noon to 4 pm: Eating

4 pm to 8 pm: Eating

8 pm to Midnight: Eating

Thursday

Midnight to 4 am: Sleeping and fasting

4 am to 8 am: Sleeping and fasting

8 am to Noon: Eating

Noon to 4 pm: Eating

4 pm to 8 pm: Eating

8 pm to Midnight: Eating

Friday

Midnight to 4 am: Sleeping and fasting

4 am to 8 am: Sleeping and fasting

8 am to Noon: Eating

Noon to 4 pm: Eating

4 pm to 8 pm: Eating

8 pm to Midnight: Eating

Saturday

Midnight to 4 am: Sleeping and fasting

4 am to 8 am: Sleeping and fasting

8 am to Noon: Eating

Noon to 4 pm: Eating

4 pm to 8 pm: Eating

8 pm to Midnight: Eating

After you successfully follow this intermittent

fasting routine, you can then try the 24-hour fast to break the mental barrier and motivate yourself to sustain it for long. It will not only provide health benefits but will motivate you to pursue it for a longer duration.

Alternate Day Fasting

As you've read, alternate day fasting is when you eat as normal on day 1, fast on day 2, eat as normal on day 3, fast on day 4, and so on. Basically, you need to eat 500 calories every alternate day in a week; this will keep your body from being overwhelmed and offer numerous health benefits. If you can, you should fast for the entire day on your alternate fasting days in a week. Begin by consuming 500 calories on your fasting day and gradually decrease it to 300 calories, 100 calories, and then 0 calories. However, this can be too stressful, so it should be followed for only a short period or not at all. You can drink water and other liquids (without sugar and additives) during this period.

To follow a weekly plan for alternate fasting more effectively, stick this schedule on your bedside table or work desk to keep track of your fasting approach for the entire week.

Sunday

Midnight to 4 am: Sleeping and fasting

4 am to 8 am: Sleeping and fasting

8 am to Noon: Eating

Noon to 4 pm: Eating

4 pm to 8 pm: Eating

8 pm to Midnight: Eating

Monday

Midnight to 4 am: Sleeping and fasting

4 am to 8 am: Sleeping and fasting

8 am to Noon: Eating

Noon to 4 pm: Eating

4 pm to 8 pm: Eating

8 pm to Midnight: Fasting

Tuesday

Midnight to 4 am: Sleeping and fasting

4 am to 8 am: Sleeping and fasting

8 am to Noon: Fasting

Noon to 4 pm: Fasting

4 pm to 8 pm: Fasting

8 pm to Midnight: Eating

Wednesday

Midnight to 4 am: Sleeping and fasting

4 am to 8 am: Sleeping and fasting

8 am to Noon: Eating

Noon to 4 pm: Eating

4 pm to 8 pm: Eating

8 pm to Midnight: Fasting

Thursday

Midnight to 4 am: Sleeping and fasting

4 am to 8 am: Sleeping and fasting

8 am to Noon: Fasting

Noon to 4 pm: Fasting

4 pm to 8 pm: Fasting

8 pm to Midnight: Eating

Friday

Midnight to 4 am: Sleeping and fasting

4 am to 8 am: Sleeping and fasting

8 am to Noon: Eating

Noon to 4 pm: Eating

4 pm to 8 pm: Eating

8 pm to Midnight: Fasting

Saturday

Midnight to 4 am: Sleeping and fasting

4 am to 8 am: Sleeping and fasting

8 am to Noon: Fasting

Noon to 4 pm: Fasting

4 pm to 8 pm: Fasting

8 pm to Midnight: Eating

Compared to the daily Leangains style of intermittent fasting, this approach provides better health benefits. However, it is one of the most uncommon and least approached fasting styles. You can try it to begin intermittent fasting for a prolonged period.

Note: these fasting schedules can be downloaded from:

https://read-2-succeed-publishing.com/

Chapter 6: Additional Tips

As you know by now, intermittent fasting can be overwhelming for most beginners. There are specific points that you should note and take care of before beginning your fasting journey.

In this chapter, we will take a look at some additional tips that will help you overcome potential issues and provide a safer way to follow this fasting approach.

1. Know When you Cannot Fast

Intermittent fasting isn't meant for just anyone. While it suits most individuals, some people with the following issues or health profile should avoid it —

• Pregnant and breastfeeding women: Since a mother and her child needs extra nutrients for the baby's growth and healthy development, pregnant and breastfeeding women should not follow intermittent fasting.

• People with a lower BMI (generally under 18.5): These individuals are considered underweight, which is why they should stay away from intermittent fasting.

• People with an eating disorder: Some people with an imbalanced BMI also face certain eating disorders, the most common being anorexia.

• Underage kids. Children below the age of 18 should not consider intermittent fasting. Teenagers are in their development phase, and they need to feed on nutrients for healthy growth.

• People who take prescription medicine.

• People suffering from type 1 or type 2 diabetes mellitus.

• If you suffer from high uric acid or gout.

• If you suffer from serious health issues, such as kidney problems, liver issues, or heart disease.

If you do not suffer from any of these issues or conditions and have stable mental health, you can definitely fast without any hindrance.

2. Stay Hydrated

Drinking plenty of water and staying hydrated all the time can seriously lower the adverse behavioral effects with intermittent fasting. When your body is in a fasted state, it might experience a loss of electrolytes and a lot of water. To avoid this, drink plenty of water daily (at least 3 to 4 liters or more) to minimize the loss of electrolytes. As mentioned, drinking water can also ward off constipation and improve your digestive system. We are already aware of the numerous health benefits of drinking water. In terms of weight loss, it prepares your body for fat burning and boosts your metabolism. If you are unable to reach the drinking water goal by the end of the day, you can use alternate methods like using a tracking or reminder app to keep you drinking water. Try to consume water with green tea or lemonade (without sugar). These drinks are low in calories and can be consumed even during the fasting window.

3. Fast on the Weekdays

To follow intermittent fasting without much hassle, you should try to do it during the weekdays, especially if you are planning to follow the 5:2 fasting approach. This approach keeps things more organized and flows smoothly with your schedule. Moreover, during weekdays, you can easily distract yourself through work and other commitments, which avoids cravings and unnecessary temptations. On the other hand, during weekends, you are usually free, and it can get difficult to birth distractions because you are always looking for something to eat. Plan your weekdays and fasting routine so that you hear yourself saying, "Wow, I did not realize that the hours went by so quickly!" or "I did not realize that I forgot to eat throughout the day."

4. Reflect on What's Worrying You

The approach of intermittent fasting can be overwhelming for beginners, especially during the initial phase. It is natural to get nervous and question everything that is thrown at you, and rightly so. However, instead of pondering on the problems, it is wiser to address them and ease your mind.

Some typical troubles and issues that worry fasting beginners.

Which meal should I skip? While some beginners are ready and delighted to skip breakfast as they never really liked eating in the morning, others are skeptical about this approach. For the latter, breakfast is the most important meal of the day, and they are unable to control their hunger in the morning. Generally, intermittent fasting is perceived as skipping breakfast and eating other meals; this increases agitation and demotivates them to follow this approach. However, as you've read so far, you can skip either your breakfast or your dinner in intermittent fasting. It doesn't matter as long as you are skipping a meal. Get this straight – breakfast is a neutral meal; eating it will do nothing special to your metabolism, and skipping it will do nothing to your weight. So, stick to an eating schedule that suits you and your routine.

Can I have snacks during the eating window? Another common misconception that floats among intermittent fasting beginners is the snack allowance. Some individuals believe that snacks should be avoided at all costs because these will increase calorie intake. In contrast, others believe that snacking is essential as it keeps you satiated and boosts metabolism. While eating snacks is entirely acceptable (unless you are binge-eating), avoiding it is also. You should only snack if you feel hungry during the eating window. If you are not hungry, do not force more calories in your body unnecessarily as it will majorly affect your calorie deficit, which is not what we want.

Will eating less reduce my metabolic rate? It is natural to assume that going without eating for longer durations can reduce the activity of your metabolism.

The approach of intermittent fasting is to make weight loss easier and not to complicate it further, which is why you should reflect on the pointers that are worrying you and find answers. There is no need to worry unnecessarily as intermittent fasting provides numerous health benefits. In fact, it is known that intermittent fasting retains more muscle during the fasting stage, burns more fat, and reduces more weight.

Conclusion

Now that you know the A to Z of intermittent fasting, it is time to begin following it.

All in all, these are some useful tips that you need to follow to survive intermittent fasting and fetch the best results from this experience.

- Keep drinking water and stay hydrated. It will help you survive the hunger pangs and avoid other issues, such as constipation.

- Experiment with different fasting windows and stick to one that works for you and provides anticipated results.

- To make fasting easier, switch to a low-carb diet between the windows; this will not only make the fasting process easier but will also boost more weight loss.

- Even though intermittent fasting offers you the flexibility of eating whatever you like, make sure that you don't binge. The last thing we want is overeating.

You are now ready to take on intermittent fasting to lose weight and gain health benefits. Best of luck to you on your weight loss journey.

If you enjoyed this book then please leave an honest review on the same Amazon page you bought it from.

Thank you!